Intermittent Fasting

The Ultimate Guide To Staying Lean And Healthy While Eating The Foods You Love!

© **Copyright 2017 - All rights reserved.**

The contents of this book may not be reproduced, duplicated or transmitted without direct written permission from the author.

Under no circumstances will any legal responsibility or blame be held against the publisher for any reparation, damages, or monetary loss due to the information herein, either directly or indirectly.

Legal Notice:
This book is copyright protected. This is only for personal use. You cannot amend, distribute, sell, use, quote or paraphrase any part or the content within this book without the consent of the author.

Disclaimer Notice:
Please note the information contained within this document is for educational and entertainment purposes only. Every attempt has been made to provide accurate, up to date and reliable complete information. No

warranties of any kind are expressed or implied. Readers acknowledge that the author is not engaging in the rendering of legal, financial, medical or professional advice. The content of this book has been derived from various sources. Please consult a licensed professional before attempting any techniques outlined in this book.

By reading this document, the reader agrees that under no circumstances are is the author responsible for any losses, direct or indirect, which are incurred as a result of the use of information contained within this document, including, but not limited to, —errors, omissions, or inaccuracies.

Free Bonus

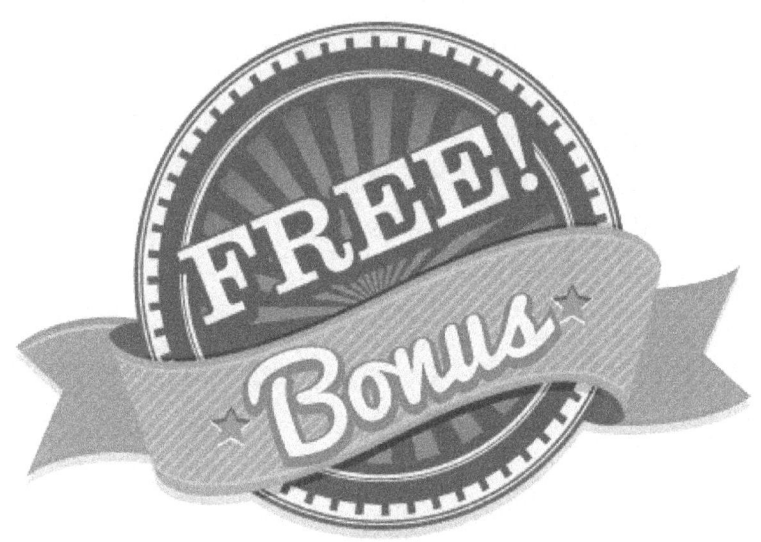

I want to thank you for purchasing this book, hence I would like to give you a free gift in return. Click here or follow the link below to claim your free gift now.
Cheers!

http://eepurl.com/cRXcDf

Table of Contents

Introduction 7
Chapter 1: Intermittent Fasting Basics 9
Chapter 2: The Lean Gains Protocol 24
Chapter 3: The Eat-Stop-Eat Protocol 28
Chapter 4: The Warrior Diet Protocol 34
Chapter 5: The Alternate Day Protocol 38
Chapter 6: The Fat Loss Forever Protocol 42
Chapter 7: The 5:2 Diet Protocol 45
Chapter 8: The Spontaneous Fasting Protocol 49
Chapter 9: Muscles – The Secret to Getting and Staying Lean 52
Chapter 10: Practical Tips for Intermittent Fasting Success 58
Chapter 11: Top Mistakes to Avoid When Fasting Intermittently 67
Conclusion 81

Introduction

There's a reason why intermittent fasting's one of the most popular eating plans in the world today: **It works!** More specifically, it helps people not just lose the right kind of weight (which you'll learn about in the book) but also become and stay healthy. While it's not a magic pill to make all your flab and sicknesses go away, it can help you achieve your ideal weight and significantly reduce your risks of certain major health conditions.

In this book, I'll show you what intermittent fasting really is, why you should incorporate it into your lifestyle, how it can help you get and stay lean and healthy, the different ways of fasting intermittently (protocols) and how to live the intermittent fasting lifestyle with a list of things you should and shouldn't do. By the time you finish reading this book, you'll be in a great position to start incorporating intermittent fasting into your lifestyle and be on your way to becoming lean and healthier.

If you're ready, turn the page and let's begin!

Chapter 1: Intermittent Fasting Basics

In order to fully understand what intermittent fasting is and why you can benefit much from it as part of your lifestyle, it's important to dissect the term into its component words – fasting and intermittent. Let's talk about fasting first.

A lot of people have many different impressions about the word "fasting." For some people, it's a diet. For some, it's a way of twisting the arm of God to get what they want from Him – as if they can twist God's arm. For some, it's a way of cleansing the body. So what is fasting, really?

Basically, fasting is the act of intentionally staying away from food for a specific period of time. A person can fast – or stay away from food – completely or partially. The reason for many people's perception about fasting as a means of obtaining the favor of God is because of its strong associations with major religions such as Christianity, Judaism and Islam. With these and other religions, fasting is one of the best ways to "please" God (whether the intention is to merely please Him or obtain His blessings), to pay for the sins they've committed, or to make their spirits stronger and more sensitive to God's voice.

The latter perception of spiritual strengthening and sharpening is surprisingly backed up by psychological principles, albeit from a different angle. How's that so?

For people who are very religious or devout, the ability to resist the world's temptations such as sex, vices and materialism, among others, is dependent on the strength of one's spirit. There's a very good spiritual analogy that illustrates the battle between the spirit and the flesh or worldly desires – the good and evil inner wolves.

The Native American Indians believe that within a person's spirit live 2 wolves, both of whom are at odds with each other. The stronger wolf is the one that makes the person think, feel and live their lives in a particular way, i.e., good or bad. And who determines who between the two wolves is stronger? The person himself.

If a person starves his fleshly wolf, the evil one, he weakens it and inadvertently feeds the good wolf to make it strong, and vice versa. Fasting is one of the major ways that most religions feed the good wolf and consequently, starve the evil one. That's why religious people believe that fasting helps strengthen the spirit, i.e., the good wolf, to fight against temptation.

In the field of psychology, the term used to refer to the practice of starving the evil wolf is delayed gratification. If you recall what happened in the now famous marshmallow test conducted on children, those who were able to resist the lure of eating the marshmallows immediately grew up to be generally well-adjusted and disciplined adults. Since fasting involves a lot of delayed gratification, it allows a person to develop a much stronger character or will power.

Why Go Hungry?

Believe it or not, the benefits of fasting aren't just limited to the spirit or the psyche. It also extends to the physical body. Now, how can going hungry for a relatively long period of time be of any physical benefit when most of what popular science says about going hungry for long periods of time isn't all that good? Further, isn't it that food is one of the essential requirements for longevity?

While it's true that food is a requirement for staying alive and hunger is generally not good for the body and mind, intentionally going hungry for a limited period of time, done the right way, can actually make a person much, much healthier both physically and mentally. The key to this is fasting intermittently, or periodically.

Which brings us to the second word of the term, which is "intermittent." The key to making the practice of intentionally going hungry a great way to achieve better health and fitness (get and stay lean) is by doing it intermittently and not for very long periods of time, i.e., for days or week on end. Doing it this way doesn't just keep you from starving excessively to the point that your health suffers, but it can actually improve your health and help you live optimally.

To be more specific, here are intermittent fasting's top health benefits:

__Accelerated Fat Loss__

Losing weight isn't necessarily a great thing, especially if you lose the wrong kind of weight. Really? There's a right kind of weight loss? You bet there is, and it's called fat loss!

Many people confuse weight loss with fat loss, which is why so many unhealthy rapid weight loss diets – a.k.a. crash diets – continue to propagate on the Internet and beyond. While it's true that many crash diets can really make a person lose 10 pounds or more per week, it's worth noting that most of such weight lost is of the kind you don't want to lose: water and muscle mass.

Intermittent fasting helps you lose the right kind of weight at a fast but healthy pace – body fat. Believe me, even if you just lose 2 pounds per week at most (the established healthy weight loss rate), 8 pounds of body fat in a month (at 4 weeks per month) will make you look significantly slimmer compared to 16 pounds in a month that's mostly water and muscle.

Why the need to preserve as much muscle mass as possible? The more muscle mass you have, the faster your metabolism is, i.e., the ability to burn calories consumed and stored body fat. When you lose mostly body fat and minimal muscle mass, your metabolism hardly changes and you'll continue burning mostly body fat the way forest fires rage through, well, forests!

Intermittent fasting helps speed up your metabolism by raising the production of fat-burning hormones such as norepinephrine while minimizing insulin production. It has been shown in studies that on average, intermittent fasting – if done right – can help your body burn up to 14% more calories and body fat. In particular, a review of a particular piece of scientific literature in 2014 showed that within 24 weeks, intermittent fasting can help people lose as much as 8% of their weight, which may be considered a substantial rate of weight loss for a relatively short period of time. Imagine if you're 200 pounds, you can lose as much as 16 pounds of mostly fat in just 6 months or less! In the same study, it was also discovered that the people who were involved in the study lost as much as 7% in terms of inches from their waistlines. This shows that most of the weight loss achieved was body fat.

In another study, intermittent fasting was shown to spare more muscle mass compared to calorie-restricted diets done over the long-term. The reason? Remember how intermittent fasting raises the production of fat-burning hormones while minimizing those of fat-inducing ones? Now you know why.

Because of its ability to limit your caloric consumption and improve your metabolism, intermittent fasting can help you achieve your weight loss, i.e., body fat loss, goals.

Minimize Type 2 Diabetes Risks

One of the world's fastest spreading health

epidemics is diabetes. In many countries the world over, especially in affluent or 1st world countries, diabetes is turning out to be one of the deadliest medical conditions that governments are battling with. This medical condition is primarily the result of heightened insulin resistance (low insulin sensitivity), which makes a person's blood sugar consistently high to the point of being chronic. Conversely, the lower a person's resistance to insulin (high sensitivity) is, the lower his or her blood sugar usually is.

As mentioned earlier, intermittent fasting can help minimize the production of insulin. In several studies, it's been estimated that intermittent fasting can bring down insulin levels by as much as 31%. In the same vein, it was also estimated based on studies that intermittent fasting can help reduce blood sugar levels by as much as 6%.

By improving insulin sensitivity (decreasing insulin resistance) and lowering your blood sugar levels, intermittent fasting can help you minimize your risks for acquiring type-2 diabetes later in life. However, this benefit is more applicable for men than women. One study showed that on average, the blood sugar levels of women increased while on a 3-week intermittent fasting protocol.

Improved Cardiovascular Health

Today, ISIS or the Syrian Army isn't the world's number one killer. It is cardiovascular diseases. And there are health markers or risk factors that can help determine one's risks of heart disease.

One of intermittent fasting's likely benefits is the reduction of some of these markers or risk factors, which include elevated cholesterol levels, hypertension, blood sugar levels, triglyceride levels and markers for inflammation. I say "likely" because these benefits were mostly observed in animal subjects, which means there's a need for more studies to be conducted – this time on humans – concerning the cardiovascular benefits of intermittent fasting. Nevertheless, the likelihood of such benefits also holding true for humans is high considering that most scientific tests on the potential effects of drugs and other things are first tested on animals. And often times, the positive test results give researchers and scientists the go signal to apply such things on humans.

Improved Cellular Restoration

One process that's crucial for cellular repair is removal of waste from the cells, i.e., **autophagy.** This involves the metabolism of dysfunctional or broken proteins, which can build up in cells over time. Increased autophagy can help metabolize or remove more of such broken or dysfunctional proteins and consequently, improve your body's cellular repair function. Intermittent fasting can help your body achieve increased autophagy and in the process, help your body repair cells much better.

Cellular, Gene, And Hormonal Changes

When you haven't had anything to eat for a meaningful length of time, several important hormonal changes happen. This includes – as mentioned earlier – increased production of the fat burning hormone norepinephrine and reduction of insulin levels. As mentioned earlier too, it also includes increased autophagy that leads to better cellular repair.

Another hormonal change that can happen while fasting intermittently is increased production of human growth hormones, which can help you build more muscle or preserve muscle mass even while dieting. Aside from making you look much fitter, more muscle mass helps you become functionally stronger.

Reduced Levels of Oxidative Stress and Inflammation

The single biggest reason for premature aging and for most chronic and degenerative health conditions today is oxidative stress. **Why?** It's because it strikes your body where it's most important – at the cellular level! Oxidative stress involves the reaction of free radicals or unstable molecules with the body's crucial molecules like protein and DNA. And such reactions aren't good – they're harmful and damaging!

It has been demonstrated in scientific studies

that intermittent fasting has the beneficial ability to help the body boost its ability to ward off or combat oxidative stress. Some studies have also revealed that intermittent fasting can also reduce another major factor for many chronic diseases: inflammation. Therefore, intermittent fasting is one of the best ways to slow down aging, and reduce your risks for many of today's chronic and **degenerative sicknesses.**

Better Management of Cancer

Some studies, albeit done on animals, have shown that intermittent fasting can help reduce risks for certain cancers through improved metabolic processes. When it comes to studies done on humans, intermittent fasting was shown to be helpful in **minimizing the side effects of chemotherapy.**

Optimal Mind

Many times, what's beneficial for the body in general is also beneficial for the brain. Better metabolism, substantial improvements in insulin and blood sugar levels, reductions in oxidative stress, and reduced inflammation can all contribute to optimal cognitive and mental performances as well as overall brain health. Animal studies have shown that intermittent fasting can help grow new nerve cells, which are crucial for optimal mental performance and brain health. Intermittent fasting has also been shown in other studies to stimulate production of brain-derived neurotropic factor (BDNF), an important hormone that can help reduce risks for mental problems like depression, among others. And lastly, intermittent fasting can also help minimize the damaging effects of strokes on one's brain.

Lower Risk for Alzheimer's disease

One of the world's most prevalent **neurodegenerative conditions** is Alzheimer's disease. Presently, there's still no known cure for Alzheimer's despite scientific breakthroughs that bring us closer to discovering such a cure. So at this point, the **best medicine is still prevention.**

While studies that have yielded significant

findings on intermittent fasting's role in lowering the risk for Alzheimer's were conducted on animals, it doesn't mean intermittent fasting's anti-Alzheimer's benefits aren't applicable to humans. Remember, most scientific breakthroughs in the medical field were first validated in animals before humans. As such, it may be the case that intermittent fasting can help reduce one's risks for Alzheimer's disease and even for Parkinson's and Huntington's diseases. And while there aren't any significant studies done on humans as of now that validates intermittent fasting's role in the war against Alzheimer's, there are reports of Alzheimer's patients experiencing much better symptoms after fasting for a short period of time as an intervention method.

Generally Longer Life

Lastly, general improvements in overall health will consequently improve one's longevity. Because intermittent fasting can help bring about the aforementioned key health and fitness benefits, it's highly likely that incorporating intermittent fasting as part of a generally healthy lifestyle can help extend one's life.

Different Strokes, Different Strokes, Same Results

There are many ways to skin a cat, as the popular saying goes. When it comes to intermittent fasting, the same applies. In the next few chapters, we'll take a look at the most popular ways intermittent fasting is done all over the world, which are more commonly referred to as protocols. Each protocol has its own unique advantages, which can help you incorporate intermittent fasting into your lifestyle regardless of your personal circumstances.

Chapter 2: The Lean Gains Protocol

This is considered to be one of the world's **most popular** protocols for fasting intermittently. The proponent of this protocol is **Martin Berkhan** and the lean gains protocol's ideal for you if you love to hit the weights at the gym and want to get ripped and shredded, i.e., build muscle and lose body fat.

How It Works

If you're a man, you will need to fast for 16 hours every day and if you're a woman, you'll need to fast for a shorter period of time daily – 14 hours. The remaining 8 (men) to 10 (women) hours will be your feeding or eating window.

You don't totally go food-less during your 14-16 hour daily fasting period. You can still eat some food during those times except that you can only eat or drink stuff that's practically calorie free. On top of the list is of course, water! Other acceptable alternatives include calorie-free sodas and gums, unsweetened black coffee (or sweetened with a calorie-free sweetener like stevia), and tea.

Next to how long will you fast on the lean gains protocol is when should you schedule it within your day? It depends really but the best time would be when it's least difficult for you to fast. For most people, their ideal fasting time is throughout the evening – it's easier to fast when asleep – until late morning. For such people, late morning is normally 6 hours upon waking up.

If you're the type of person who has very hectic days most of the time, timing your eating window so that it corresponds to your days' busiest or most hectic times can help provide you with the necessary energy when you need it most. And scheduling your fasting period on your most "down" times will help you hold on to your fast.

More than just eating and not eating, you will also need to pay close attention to what you should and shouldn't eat during your feeding windows. In particular, you will need to consider that kinds of foods that are optimal for your regular workouts at the gym. On the days you'll be hitting the gym, you'll need more carbohydrates for fuel and less fat calories. But on days you won't be hitting the gym, more fat calories than carbs is better. **Why?** Fat calories are more satiating, i.e., more filling, which can help you feel fuller for longer and reduce your cravings or hunger during your fasting window. But regardless of whether or not you hit the gym, you must make sure to include adequate amounts of protein for muscle sparing or building.

Regardless of the type of calorie you'll be eating, it's important to eat whole and unprocessed foods most of the time. Once in a while, there's no harm in going for processed ones like a meal replacement shake or a granola bar, especially when you're in a tight fix. Just make sure that eating processed foods remain to be the exception rather than the norm.

Pros and Cons

As with all good things, this protocol has its own set of advantages and disadvantages. Let's talk about advantage first, foremost of which is that there'll be no fuss concerning the frequency of meals. Whether you eat everything in one sitting or 20 sittings, it doesn't matter as long as you eat within your designated feeding window only. For many people, the leeway to decide on how frequently to eat on a given day is a great blessing that allows them to really stick to intermittent fasting.

What the protocol gives by way of total freedom in choosing meal frequencies is often negated or mitigated by its relatively "strict" guideline on what types of calories to consume on a given day, i.e., more carbs than fat on workout days and more fats than carbs on non-workout days. For some people, this is quite cumbersome and thus, they fail to stick to the protocol altogether.

Chapter 3: The Eat-Stop-Eat Protocol

This intermittent fasting protocol was created by a dude named **Brad Pilon.** If you're the type of person who's already eating right and healthy, then this may be the protocol for you. Compared to some of the relatively extreme eating protocols, the eat-stop-eat protocol's primarily hinged on moderation. What do I mean by that?

Here, you can eat pretty much anything you like for as long as you only eat moderate amounts of such. So if you want to eat a slice of pizza, go ahead! Just make sure you stick to that slice only and leave the rest of the other slices alone.

How It Works

With the eat-stop-eat method, you don't need to fast everyday. You'll only have to do it at most twice weekly for 24 hours each time.

And during those 24-hour fasting periods, you can't eat anything but you may freely drink any beverage for as long as it doesn't have calories, e.g., water and green tea.

When your fasting period's done, you simply go back to your usual eating program. And according to the protocol's creator Brad Pilon, you can live as if you never fasted at all. With such leeway, different people break their fasts differently. Some just eat normally while others binge eat with one humongous meal. Still others do so by just enjoying a light snack. It's really up to you how you'd like to break your weekly fasts.

You also have the liberty of choosing the timing of your weekly fast or fasts. This means you can schedule your fast or fasts on days when you know you'll have the least difficult time fasting for 24 hours. For some people, it's the weekends while for some, it's when they're most busy at work so that they hardly become mindful of their being hungry. It's really up to you.

As mentioned earlier, this protocol's all about moderation. As such, it is one that aims to reduce your caloric consumption by reducing your meal frequency for the whole week, i.e., not eating for 1 or 2 days every week. By doing so, it inadvertently reduces your weekly caloric intake en route to fat loss.

Regular exercise is another important part of this particular protocol. In terms of such, weight lifting or resistance training exercises are the best ones to regularly perform. Why? It's because weight-training exercises are the best for at least maintaining or minimizing muscle mass loss while losing weight. And as I mentioned earlier, muscle mass is one of the most important factors that will determine how much calories your body can burn regularly and how much body fat you can lose while dieting.

Pros and Cons

When it comes to the Eat-Stop-Eat protocol, its biggest advantage is flexibility. Why? It's because this protocol lets you start small and take initially small but ever increasing steps towards full implementation. What this means is you don't need to put it all on the line and implement the protocol fully on your first day, which can be hard, especially when you haven't fasted your whole life. You can start by fasting for as long as you possibly can during the first day or two and gradually increasing the duration of your regular fasts as your body responds accordingly.

Brad Pilon – the protocol's creator and chief proponent – espouses that you start doing the protocol on your week's potentially busiest day or on a day where you don't have social gathering commitments to fulfill (minimize food temptations). By starting the protocol on a day that's characterized by at least one of the 2 conditions, you may be able to keep your mind too preoccupied to be conscious of food (or the lack of it), minimize the temptation to break your fast too early, or both.

Another **key benefit** of the protocol is that there is neither forbidden food items nor a duty to watch your calories like Golden State Warriors fans keep tabs on Steph Curry's 3-point shots made for the season. The fact that you don't need to strictly monitor what and how much you eat makes it substantially less difficult to implement this protocol compared to many other intermittent fasting methods. But nevertheless, it's important to keep in mind that this protocol isn't a license to buffet everyday like it's the end of the world. The key – as to anything else – is moderation. Eat anything you want but remember not to overdo it.

As for disadvantages, the only one associated with the Eat-Stop-Eat protocol is the duration of the fast, which is at least 24 hours. Whether, once or twice a week only, 24 hours without food can still be very challenging for most people especially during the first several weeks of implementation of the protocol, where side effects can be experienced. These can include being cranky, headaches, fatigue, or anxiety, which eventually fade away after the first several weeks.

If you choose to implement this protocol, know that the **24-hour** fast is a very challenging one, even if you gradually build up your fasting duration towards it. As such, the temptation to binge eat every time you break the fast can be very powerful. This is where you'll need to exert every ounce of willpower that you have to make sure you eat moderately when breaking your fasts under this protocol.

Chapter 4: The Warrior Diet Protocol

As the name suggests, this protocol requires you to eat like a **"warrior"**. And what does it mean to eat like one? For sure, it's not eating like the Golden State Warriors.

The protocol's creator, **Ori Hofmekler,** believes that warriors from the ancient times – particularly those training to be such – eat just 1 big meal everyday, which is dinner. For the rest of the 24 daily hours, these warriors fast. This particular protocol will suit you well if you're the type of person who is devoted to rules or a stickler for such.

How It Works

The diet is a **very simple one** – eat one large meal a day at night. That's it. Very simple isn't it? But why schedule your one big meal at night, which is contrary to what many conventional nutritional experts say?

It's because according to Hofmekler, humans are naturally nocturnal or night eaters by genetic design. Given this particular genetic trait, it only makes sense to schedule your 1 big meal at night so that you can optimally feed your body with all the nutrients it needs as your body's circadian or sleep rhythm requires. Hofmekler explains that the reason for such is that doing so helps increase your parasympathetic nervous system's capacity to help your body relax, digest your food, recuperate, and calm down, all of which are conducive for maximum cellular repair and growth.

Further, Hofmekler claims that eating just one big meal in the evening can also help your body produce key hormones and consequently, burn more body fat during daytime. And when doing so, you will also need to consider the order by which you eat certain types of food during your 4-hour nighttime eating window. He recommends that you eat your veggies first, proteins next, and fats for last. And if despite your single big meal you're still hungry, you can eat some more carbs.

From the perspective of the Warrior Diet protocol, fasting is about eating below your means versus starvation. This perspective then allows you to actually eat during your fasting period, only that you eat small portions or servings of fruits, raw veggies, fresh juice, or protein. Doing this can help you boost your energy, optimize fat burning, and increase mental alertness throughout the day while fasting by increasing or boosting your sympathetic nervous system's flight-or-fight response.

Pros and Cons

The Warrior Diet protocol's main advantage is that technically speaking, it isn't a fast because it allows you to eat small portions of raw veggies, fruits, proteins, and juices during your 20-hour daily fasting period. As mentioned earlier, it's really more about under-eating more than starving yourself, which is what fasts are all about. This can make it much easier for you to implement consistently and stay on for the long term.

Other reported advantages of this protocol include significant improvements in energy levels and ability to burn body fat.

While the diet seems much easier to implement given you won't be starving yourself throughout your daily fasting periods of up to 20 hours, it can be challenging in terms of permitted foods to eat and eating schedule. Because you will be limited to veggies, lean proteins and good dietary fat and you can only eat a meal in the evening, it can prove to be rather challenging to attend most social gatherings while keeping strict compliance with the protocol.

Another potential disadvantage, particularly in the beginning, is the difficulty of eating practically all of your daily caloric requirements in the evening in just one sitting. This can be more pronounced considering most people are used to eating most of their daily food requirements during the day. But over time, this can be less challenging, as you gradually grow **accustomed to nocturnal eating.**

Chapter 5: The Alternate Day Protocol

This protocol was created by **Dr. James Johnson, MD.** Compared to the other intermittent fasting protocols, the Alternate Day diet may be considered one of the **easier protocols** to implement. It's because the protocol only requires you to fast every other day, i.e., you eat very little on your fasting days and eat normally in between days.

How It Works

It's worth clarifying what eating "very little" means because let's face it, the term means different things to different people. For **Shaquille O'Neal,** who stands 7 feet 1 inch tall and weighs 324 pounds, the term "very little" may already be considered as a buffet for Isaiah Thomas who stands just 5 feet 9 inches and weighs just a little over 185 pounds. So for purposes of this protocol, "very little" means getting just 20% of your daily caloric requirements or consumption. So if you're usually consuming **2,500 calories** a day, you only consume **500 calories** on your fasting days.

For convenience's sake, Dr. Johnson suggests drinking meal replacement shakes on the days that you fast. It's because such shakes can be easily consumed throughout the day and they can pack a lot of nutrients. But Dr. Johnson doesn't favor dependence on it. He says that past the first **2 weeks** of your starting the protocol, you must go back to eating real, whole foods during your fasting days.

And remember how we talked about regular weight lifting exercise being part of the warrior diet protocol? Weight lifting exercises are also a crucial part of the Alternate Day protocol. Because of that, the best time to schedule your workouts is on the days that you don't fast. Doing so will help you exert maximum effort doing your workouts and make the most out of them.

Pros and Cons

The alternate day protocol is one that's primarily focused on helping you lose the healthy kind of weight, which is body fat. If you lose more body fat than water or muscle mass in terms of weight, you won't just look and feel fit. You'll also be much healthier. Based on Dr. Johnson's website, you can lose as much as **2.5 pounds** weekly, which is what most health and fitness experts consider to be a safe weight loss pace.

Another advantage of this protocol is its relative simplicity. No calorie counting or having to watch what you eat. It's one less stress on your mind.

But its relative simplicity can also be a disadvantage in that you severely cut your calories every other day to only **20%** of your usual, which can be too much if you're not used to fasting. While it may be simple to practically eat nothing the whole day every other day, it's not the easiest thing in the world to do. And it's higher than normal level of difficulty can make your risks for binge eating on normal days much higher. That's unless you have a very strong will power or you can effectively plan your activities far ahead in advance to ensure that you minimize temptations for eating more than that which is required on both your fasting and normal eating days.

Chapter 6: The Fat Loss Forever Protocol

This intermittent fasting protocol was developed by **Dan Go** and **John Romaniello.** If you're a gym rat who thinks of diet cheat days as God's greatest gift to gym rats, then this protocol may be the ideal one for you. Why?

One reason is that it brings together the best of the Lean Gains, Eat-Stop-Eat, and Warrior Diet protocols in just one. Think of it as a pack of 3-in-1 coffee only that it's intermittent fasting.

Two of its major features is a push and pull sort of relationship between heaven and hell, where you get 1 whole day for cheat meals every week (heaven) followed by a 36-hour fast (hell). The 5 other days are then divided among the 3 different protocols according to your preference.

The protocols creators suggest that you schedule your longest fasting period on the days that you're busiest. Why? So that your mind will be too preoccupied to think about or notice the hunger that's brewing in your stomach. You can buy the protocol's plan on Dan and John's website and get free training programs (bodyweight and free weight exercises), which can help you make the most out of your healthy weight loss (fat loss) efforts.

Pros and Cons

Its most significant pro is that the **7-day** cycle for fasting lets your body acclimatize to a fasting table that has a structure. As a result, you can maximize the fat burning and muscle-building results of the protocol and your training program. Per Dan and John, everybody fasts on a daily basis. The only difference is how they do it, e.g., others do it carelessly. With the Fat Loss Forever protocol, you can fast in a highly structured, controlled, and effective manner.

Its disadvantage? Well, it's similar to the other protocols in that after the longest fast of the week, i.e., **36 hours,** the temptation to binge eat as you break that fast is very high compared to other protocols given that you fasted for a significantly longer period of time.

Another potential disadvantage of the protocol – at least at first – is that it can be quite confusing or challenging to follow strictly. Why? It's because of its strict but widely varying schedules throughout the 7-day cycle. Remember that for **5** days, you'll be doing the 3 protocols we mentioned earlier, which can keep you from establishing a rhythm or pattern. But as you progress along with the protocol, you'll eventually get used to it.

Chapter 7: The 5:2 Diet Protocol

Also referred to as **The Fast Diet,** the 5:2 protocol is one of the most, if not the most, popular of the intermittent fasting protocols these days. Why?

How It Works

The protocol – made popular by British journalist and **Doctor Michael Mosley** – lets people eat normally for 5 days in a week and fast for only 2 days. Now you may be wondering, isn't this how the Eat-Stop-Eat method works? On the surface, it seems so. But actually, they work differently.

For one, you can fast just one day during the week with the Eat-Stop-Eat protocol while under the 5:2 protocol, you fast for 2 days. Another key difference is that you can actually eat during the 2 fasting days under the 5:2 protocol while in the Eat-Stop-Eat method, you can only enjoy calorie free drinks while fasting.

Speaking of calories, you're allowed to consume a total of **500 calories** if you're a woman or **600 calories** if you're a man on your fasting days. There are no "rules" as to what you can and can't eat or when you should eat during your fasting days. But if you want to minimize the stress, you can follow the lead of many people who've already done the 5:2 Diet protocol, which is to follow one of the 2 fasting patterns:
- Three (3) mini-meals, one each over breakfast, lunch, and dinner; or
- Two (2) smaller than normal meals, normally over lunch and dinner.

Remember that the only rule here is to limit caloric intake to a maximum of **600** and **500** calories if you're a man or a woman, respectively, throughout your fasting day. Therefore, you should budget your calories wisely across the day.

While there's no "right" or "wrong" foods under this protocol, there are wise and unwise choices. Going for food items that are high in fiber and protein are generally wise choices as these help you feel full for longer and can significantly reduce hunger pangs. In turn, those can help you keep your calories to within the daily limit.

Another wise food choice are soups made from whole food ingredients. Don't go for commercially available and synthetic "instant" soups. They're neither good for your health nor your waistline.

The only other rule you'll need to abide by under this protocol is to ensure that there's at least 1 normal eating day in between your **2** days of weekly fasting. Many people who do this protocol schedule their fasting days every Monday and Thursday, eating **3** small meals on each of those days, and eating normally for the remaining days.

And speaking of eating normally, please don't confuse it with "buffet" or eating as much as you can. Normally means just that, normal. Eat the same amount as you normally would when you're not fasting.

Pros and Cons

One of the advantages of this protocol is that it doesn't really feel like a diet because it's more an eating pattern than a "fast". Not only do you get to eat small portions of food on your fasting days, which is only for 2 days every week, but you also have no restrictions as to the kinds of foods to eat. As such, many people feel it's much easier to stick to this protocol than most other intermittent fasting protocols or weight loss diets for that matter.

The only **disadvantage of this protocol** in my viewpoint is that you won't lose as much weight as most of the others given it's more lenient in terms of caloric consumption. Your fasting days are more like "severe calorie restriction" days rather than non-eating days. But if you feel you're not hardcore enough to lose more weight on the other harder protocols, it's alright. To each his own and if this protocol suits you best, then by all means go for it.

Chapter 8: The Spontaneous Fasting Protocol

The last protocol we'll be looking at is what I'd consider to be Intermittent Fasting Lite because it's the **easiest of all protocols.** Why?

How It Works

As the name suggests, there are no rules as to when you'll fast. Fasting under this protocol is pretty much like watching movies on **Netflix,** i.e., on demand. Here, you won't have to stick to a particular structure for fasting intermittently. You just fast on the go and off the fly! Just skip meals every now and then, especially when you're not hungry yet or have so much to do that you can't afford to eat. Just make sure you get to eat nutritious and healthy meals when you do decide to eat.

In a nutshell, the spontaneous fasting protocol is a more organic way of fasting intermittently by skipping one or 2 meals daily when it's most convenient.

Pros and Cons

Obviously, its greatest advantage is the lack of structure. You can skip your meals at your most convenient times of the day and there are no forbidden foods. As such, there's really no reason for you not to be able to fast intermittently except for one: you don't really want to do it.

Its greatest advantage can also be its biggest disadvantage. Some people need structure in order to get things done and if you're such a person, the lack of structure of this diet can make it hard for you to successfully implement it.

Another disadvantage of this intermittent fasting protocol is that being the easiest one to do, it may also reap the least beneficial results, especially when it comes to healthy weight loss. Let's face it, healthy weight loss is still all about calorie reduction and being in a consistent state of caloric deficits, i.e., calories consumed are less than calories used or burned. A protocol that's not predicated on any consistent effort for significantly reducing calories is one that may keep you from optimal weight or fat loss. It's either you lose significant weight much longer than the other protocols or you lose significantly less weight for a given period of time compared to the other protocols. Such is the trade-off between convenience and results.

Chapter 9: Muscles – The Secret to Getting and Staying Lean

When it comes to healthy weight loss, i.e., body fat loss, nutrition or diet is just part of the equation. Another crucial aspect – maybe an even more important one – is metabolism or the rate at which your body's able to burn calories or body fat. Obviously, the higher your metabolism is, the more calories or body fat your body can burn. So a fast metabolism coupled with calorie reduction is a potent one-two punch against body fat.

And when it comes to metabolism, one of the most important factors affecting it is the amount of muscle mass your body has. Why? Of all your body's cells, muscles are the most metabolically active, i.e., require the most calories for normal functioning. It therefore follows that the more muscle mass you have, the faster your metabolism can be and consequently, your metabolism slows down when your muscle mass is reduced.

When it comes to maintaining or even increasing muscle mass while fasting intermittently, there's a lot of "passionate" discussions going around. Many who take the conventional point of view say that severe caloric restriction – as is the case when fasting – leads to breaking down of muscle tissue and consequently, to muscle loss. But just how true are statements like these?

To answer that question, we'll need to consider 2 things. First is the kind of calories you consume. The second is the timing of the consumption, i.e. when you eat them. The following practical tips will help you address these 2 factors in ways that will allow you to maintain or even increase muscle mass even while fasting intermittently.

Eat Breakfast

Whether as a means by which to break your fast or a way to begin it, aim to eat something in the morning according to your chosen fasting schedule. If you choose to fast at night, then break your fast in the day with a – pardon the pun – small breakfast to launch your day on an energized note. If you choose to fast during the day, do the same, i.e., eat a small breakfast just before your fasting period begins to start the day somewhat energized as well.

But considering that you want to keep an optimal metabolism through muscle mass, building or maintaining muscle mass must be your primary focus or priority. And whether you choose to fast during the day or all throughout the night, one great way to keep your muscles well-nourished and primed up for growth or maintenance is by eating something the moment you wake up.

So what's the best food to eat in the morning for optimal muscle maintenance or growth? As much as possible, go for proteins that are slow to digest such as cheese, red meat, and eggs. **Why?** More than just making you feel satiated for much longer, they provide your muscles with the primary building blocks for growth or maintenance – protein. And aside from protein, you'll also benefit from eating some carbohydrates as it can help your mental and physical performance during the day.

When it comes to the timing of your fasting period, there's only 1 significant difference, which is the ability to spread out your caloric consumption. If you fast in the evening, you can spread out your caloric consumption throughout the full range of your eating window because you're awake. If you choose to fast during the day, you only get to eat your total calories for the 24-hour period in one big meal at night. That's unless you fancy waking up in the middle of the night to spread out your daily caloric consumption over several meals.

Schedule Your Workouts Later In the Day

Before you hit the weights, or perform bodyweight exercises such as **plyometrics or calisthenics,** it's paramount that you're able to get in a significant amount of calories in order to perform your exercises well and not faint from exhaustion. And hitting the gym, or doing calisthenics or plyometrics later in the day can help you do those regardless if you choose to fast during the day or night.

If you go for daytime fasting that ends late in the afternoon or early evening, say at 6 p.m., it will do you well to schedule your workouts later in the evening after you've gotten the chance to eat something. Aside from having enough energy, working out later in the evening increases your odds of using the machines you fancy as most people would've been done with their workouts, leaving you with very little competition for gym equipment.

If you choose to fast at night, working out late in the afternoon or early evening's your best bet. So if you start your fast at 5 or 6 in the afternoon, your best bet for working out is at 4 or 5 p.m., respectively. Doing so gives you just the opportunity to get your final calories in before and immediately after your workout just prior to starting your fasting period.

You may think, why not work out in the middle of the day? It's not a good idea especially if you fast during the day because you won't have the opportunity to get enough calories in for a meaningful workout. If you choose to work out in the morning, it'll be too cumbersome especially if you have a day job.

Eat After Working Out

Lastly, you should do your best to schedule the consumption of the bulk of your daily calories immediately after your workouts. Why? It's because of what's referred to as the **2-hour golden post-workout window** wherein your body's ability to recover and build muscle can be maximized via immediate post-workout nutrients. And more importantly, your body's chances of storing all those extra calories from post-workout meals are at its lowest during this golden window because your body, particularly your muscles, need all the protein it can get for rebuilding and all the carbohydrates it can get to quickly replenish its glycogen stores, i.e., it's primary fuel. And eating too much just before working out increases your chances of feeling lethargic and sluggish while exercising.

Chapter 10: Practical Tips for Intermittent Fasting Success

Make no mistake about it, intermittent fasting is one of the most effective method for getting into the best shape of your life and improving your health. However, it's not something that works for everyone, i.e., a one-size-works-for-all thing. For some people, intermittent fasting may even be detrimental to their health if they have pre-existing chronic sicknesses, medical issues, or special dietary needs. If you're one of them, it's best to check with your doctor first to see if intermittent fasting won't be harmful to you given your medical condition or unique dietary needs.

Assuming that you're generally healthy and have no special nutritional requirements, you must be very sensitive to the signals your body may give if you decide to fast intermittently. You must be able to sense if your body's legitimately screaming for help and get appropriate medical help, or if it's just complaining about how uncomfortable intermittent fasting is during the first few weeks. Let's face it – most people don't consider intermittent fasting "normal" and because of that, it will really take some time to acclimatize to the lifestyle. And for women, volatile hormonal levels can make it much more challenging to start and stay on any intermittent fasting protocol compared to men.

When it comes to intermittent fasting, you're better off being prudent by being careful or cautious in the beginning and gradually transitioning from short periods of fasting to much longer durations. If despite your best efforts and several weeks into the lifestyle you still feel very uncomfortable, there's no shame in accepting that intermittent fasting may not be for you and that other nutritional approaches may be your thing. Not being able to fast intermittently as a lifestyle won't erode your value as a person.

In order to maximize your chances of successfully transitioning to the intermittent fasting lifestyle, consider the following practical tips for starting the lifestyle.

Water

While you're in a fasting phase or period, one of the most – if not the most – important things you'll need is water. Unfortunately, many people who are into the intermittent fasting lifestyle are frequently dehydrated. And being frequently dehydrated while on any intermittent fasting protocol is bad for you. Why?

Your body is primarily made up of water. Yes, up to 70% of your body's made up of the stuff and as such, substantial drops in your body's water levels can have subtle but substantial impact on your cells and nerves that can impede optimal mental and physical performance.

Chronic dehydration can also make you susceptible to dizziness, constipation, dry skin, and fatigue, among others. And when you're fasting, you should stick to drinking pure water for hydration because anything else may contain high amounts of sugar and hidden calories, even if the labels say "sugar free" or "zero calories".

Another reason why you need to get enough water for healthy weight loss while fasting intermittently regardless of your chosen protocol is that it helps you feel fuller for longer. That's why even during the night, it's important that you still get to drink a glass or two of water, particularly when you're fasting. It helps you minimize hunger pangs.

So how much water is enough water? It's best to get more than **8 glasses daily** since you're fasting intermittently, and even more importantly if you're exercising regularly. And make sure that you spread out your water over several drinks throughout the day and night instead of just one or two drinks. Believe me, drinking your daily water requirements in just one or two sittings can be very uncomfortable to do regularly.

While drinking very cold water is very refreshing especially on hot days or nights, you'd be better off drinking room temperature or slightly cold water. **Why?** It's because very cold water can stimulate contraction in your blood vessels and cause indigestion.

The foods you choose to eat within your feeding windows may also impact your hydration levels. One of the foods you should minimize or avoid altogether are spicy ones because of their tendency to make you much thirstier. Salt is an ingredient that can make you significantly thirstier than usual so keep your consumption of very salty food to a minimum. And if you do eat very salty food, make sure to increase your water intake in order to lessen the relatively strong taste.

You can increase your chances of being adequately hydrated by eating fruits and veggies that are fibrous and loaded with water. More than just helping you with hydration, they also have the effect of making you feel fuller for longer.

And if you want to enjoy a glass or two of fruit juice, don't go for commercially available ones, no matter how much manufacturers claim them to be **"all natural"**. Truth is, commercially available fruit juices are laden with sugar so you're best bet is to drink freshly squeezed or pressed fruit juice. That way, you can be 100% sure that what you're drinking doesn't contain excess sugar or other harmful ingredients.

Scheduling Your Fast

The timing of your fasting periods can be a significant factor in terms of you being able to do intermittent fasting long enough to experience its benefits. This can be even more crucial if you choose to maximize fat loss through regular workouts at the gym.

Many people who fast intermittently have day jobs and other big responsibilities to take care of. That's why for them, choosing the optimal time for their fasting phases is of prime importance. That's why most people tend to schedule their fasting periods throughout the evening and into the morning. By doing so, they're able to feed themselves when they need to the most, which is during the day, and fast when energy expenditure's lowest, i.e., throughout the night. So if you're seriously considering getting into the intermittent fasting lifestyle, consider timing your fasts in the evening, where the risk of breaking your fast prematurely is at its lowest.

Lift Weights

Exercise that's called by any other name – contrary to popular notion – will neither burn the same amount of body fat nor make you look healthy and fit. That's why in case you still haven't noticed, I keep on promoting weight lifting or resistance exercises, including calisthenics and plyometrics, as the primary mode of regular exercise. And again, the reason behind it is that resistance or weight lifting exercises are best for both burning fat and building muscle.

I've seen friends who only dieted without exercising and when they lost weight, they look like they contracted some serious sickness. While they lost weight, they didn't look fit. They looked weak and frail because most of their weight loss was water and worse, muscle mass.

Contrast it to my friends and myself who have lost some weight but looked as fit as hell. How'd that happen despite not losing as much "weight" as my pure-diet-friends? It's because while we lost much body fat, we also gained muscle mass, which kind of ate into the total weight loss figure. That's why despite losing less pounds than my pure-diet friends, we looked like we lost more weight and looked much fitter and stronger.

And when it comes to resistance or weight lifting exercises, please don't think you need to be a power lifter or bodybuilder, or perform their grueling workouts. Those guys and gals are extreme and chances are, your body won't be able to handle it. All you need to do is perform basic compound lifts such as deadlifts, bench presses, and squats using enough weight where you reach failure, i.e., can no longer lift the weight, for a 9th straight repetition. Do **3 sets of 8 reps** max for each weight lifting exercise for optimal muscle training.

If you don't have access to a gym or a set of weights, you can perform bodyweight exercises such as plyometrics and calisthenics instead. Your body is a good weight to work with. Start with the number of reps you can do for each exercise and gradually build up to

12 reps per set, going for at least 2 sets per exercise.

Chapter 11: Top Mistakes to Avoid When Fasting Intermittently

Doing things right is just half the battle. The other half is avoiding mistakes that can derail your success, especially the crucial ones. And when it comes to intermittent fasting for weight, loss, health, and energy, it's the same. That's why in this final chapter, we'll discuss the top mistakes that can keep you from succeeding at intermittent fasting and how to avoid them.

Eating the Wrong Foods

Many folks who claim to have faithfully complied with intermittent fasting's guidelines and protocols don't have the bodies to show for it. Why's that so, considering they've reportedly stuck to their fasting and eating windows like bubble gum sticks to hair? If you ask them what they normally eat during their feeding windows, you'd be shocked to hear their answers: they eat mostly processed and junk foods.

There's a saying that garbage in, garbage out. When it comes to getting into great shape and health, nothing else is as true. What you eat will ultimately determine how you look and feel. No intermittent fasting protocol will ever cut it for you if you eat like crap.

Yes, there are a few very gifted people who seem to be exempted from this curse of garbage-eat-garbage-body. And they're the very few exceptions to the rule. So don't for one second take for granted that you're one of them. Unless there's compelling evidence that you are, you're not. You should take great care in choosing the foods you will regularly eat and you shouldn't leave your diet to chance.

So how does it look like to eat healthy? For one, healthy eating means eating mostly whole or "natural" foods, i.e., foods that are as close to their original states as possible. The more processed a food is, i.e., the farther it looks from its original form, the more unhealthy ingredients have been added to them, many of which won't just keep you fat but also make you sick over the long term.

So how do whole foods look like? Grilled chicken, steak, and pork chops are natural or whole foods because they haven't changed from their original form. On the other hand, burgers, hotdogs, and chicken nuggets are some of the best examples of processed foods, the consumptions of which you must minimize for health and fitness purposes. Other examples of highly processed foods are bagels, donuts, cookies...and the list goes on!

Another type of food you must minimize or even avoid altogether are sugar-filled foods and drinks. Not only are these calorie dense, i.e., pack a lot of calories for little volume, they also put you at risk for screwed up metabolism and diabetes. Stick to pure water, green tea or unsweetened coffee for drinks and fruits, veggies, and brown rice for carbs instead.

So Much Free Time

There's a saying that idle hands are the devil's

workshop. In a practical sense, it's true because when you have so much time on your hands, you will tend to fill it up with anything that's within reach. It's because people aren't wired to do nothing – we'll always look for something to fill up our time with. And often times, the most proximate or convenient way to fill up vacant time is through sedentary activities and food. Worse, junk and processed foods are the most convenient types around.

In order to avoid falling into this trap, I'm not suggesting that you fill up each and every second of your free time and refuse to have much needed down time. The keyword here is excessive because beyond what you really need for regular rest and relaxation lie the strongest temptations for all things unhealthy and fattening.

One of the best ways to minimize your risks for falling into this trap is to begin your intermittent fasting on a day that you perceive will be a very busy one. When you do that, your mind will be too preoccupied with all the things you need to do to the point that it won't be as conscious of the substantial dietary changes involved. If you start your intermittent fasting journey on a lazy day at home, your risk for breaking the fast prematurely on the first day is high because most if not all of your attention will be focused on nothing else but your hunger.

Overdosing On Stimulants

Caffeine's been scientifically proven to help optimize physical and mental performance by, among others, increasing your heart rate and making you feel awake. As a result, it can also help you burn more body fat when fasting intermittently.

But while it can be a great thing, all things good or great can be detrimental once taken excessively. A cup or two of your favorite unsweetened black coffee or green tea can be very helpful during the day, but drinking 3 or more on a regular basis isn't. Because of its acidic nature, drinking excessive caffeine can make you feel much hungrier than you really are and make it really hard for you to stay on your fast.

Too much caffeine will also rob you of a great night's rest, which is even more important if you're fasting intermittently. Lack of quality sleep will make you feel weak, sluggish, and hazy during the day, all of which substantially increases your risk for overcompensation with – you guessed it right – food! As a good general guideline, your last cup should be at 3 in the afternoon at the latest. That should give your body enough time to flush out the caffeine from your system so you can get a great night's sleep.

Setting Goals That Are Too Lofty

One way that you can fail even before you start fasting intermittently is by setting unrealistic goals for yourself on your fast. When you do that, you're merely setting yourself up to fail big time. And such hard failures can knock the wind out of you to the point that you'd want to ditch intermittent fasting altogether.

When aiming to achieve personal goals, the wise thing to do is set smaller, more realistic goals that build up towards your major ones. But these goals need to be challenging as well.

Why? If they're not challenging, accomplishing them won't mean anything to you and that means you won't be encouraged to aim for the next higher ones. If you set smaller, realistic and challenging goals, you set yourself up to experience small but major victories that will build up your confidence in achieving bigger goals.

How does this look like for intermittent fasting? Instead of aiming to be able to fast 16 hours straight, make it your first goal to skip 1 major meal a day, i.e., lunch, or dinner. If that's too big for you, try skipping snacks first before going to the major meals. That way, you don't shock your body by going cold turkey on food. And by gradually building up the duration of your fasting periods, you get to build up your capacity and confidence to fast for substantially longer periods of time.

Another example is weight loss. If you need to lose a total of 50 pounds, don't make it your goal to lose 50 pounds right off the bat. Start by making it your goal to lose 10 pounds over 2 months first. Once you get that out of the way, aim for the next 10 pounds, and so on until you eventually reach 50 pounds.

Fear of the Empty Stomach

The biggest fear of many dieters, especially those who want to embrace the intermittent fasting lifestyle, is the fear of going hungry as if it's the devil's child. Hunger is nothing but another part of normal, everyday living and unlike what many nutrition and fitness "gurus" preach, intermittent fasting won't lead to muscle wastage or loss if done right. You also won't die prematurely after fasting for 24 hours unless you've been fasting for 30 days already!

As mentioned in Chapter 1, purposefully going hungry through proper intermittent fasting protocols can actually be very beneficial for your health and overall fitness. If intermittent fasting is a sure way to shrivel your muscles away and die from hunger, why does regular or intermittent fasting play a major part in the lives of millions of people all over the world who still happen to be alive, alert, awake, and enthusiastic?

Continuously going hungry for excessive

periods of time is unhealthy or even downright dangerous. But that's not what intermittent fasting is. The word "intermittent" means among other things sporadic, irregular, or erratic. In other words, intermittent implies something that's not continuous or long lasting. It's a stop-and-go thing. By going hungry intermittently, you won't go to the extreme of starving to death.

Being Overly Cautious

There's an important principle in finance – particularly investments – that may also be applied to intermittent fasting. It says that if you want to earn higher returns or profits, you'll need to take higher risks or more volatility. And according to Mr. Hofmekler (remember him of the Warrior Diet fame?), volatility is your best friend when it comes to effective intermittent fasting. To cut all the technical mumbo-jumbo, Hofmekler claims that the nutrients you consume or ingest become even more beneficial or powerful if your body doesn't get them regularly, i.e., consumption is unpredictable. When you start to fast intermittently, you actually break the predictable nutrient consumption pattern that your body's been used to for practically your whole life. And with such unpredictability comes greater results.

Looking at "hunger" in a negative light can make you overly cautious and avoid it at all costs. But as with investments, you'll need to take bolder, riskier steps if you want to achieve greater returns. In this case, you will need to put down some of your personal walls that can keep you from embracing sporadically purposeful hunger as your ally. By taking the risk of intentionally going hungry, you'll break your body's predictable feeding pattern and in the process, you'll significantly increase the nutritional benefits it gets from the foods you'll eat.

Much Ado about Timelines

No doubt about it – the duration of your fast and how you time them are important aspects of intermittent fasting. But that doesn't mean you should be obsessed with timing because being so can just stress you out and negate or mitigate your chances of successfully achieving your fitness and health goals through intermittent fasting. You should take it seriously, no doubt about it, but you shouldn't overdo it. You must also learn how to relax.

So how can you tell if you're obsessed about timelines? If you easily get stressed over instances when you aren't able to fast or feed at your appointed "right" times, then you probably are. While you should do your best to stick to your appointed feasting and fasting periods, being off by minutes won't derail your efforts to lose body fat and achieve great health.

Looking At Individual Components Instead Of the Overall Picture

The word synergy implies that the whole is greater than the sum of its parts. Now what does that mean in layman's terms? With synergy, 5 plus 5 equals 15! Without synergy, or using the simple arithmetic method, 5 plus 5 is just 10, which is the sum of its parts.

When it comes to intermittent fasting, the beneficial results are due to the synergistic interactions of its different aspects.

Intermittent fasting doesn't work on a per aspect or component basis – they work as a team. It's a holistic endeavor. Focusing on just one or two components, e.g., fasting, feeding, or hydration, won't get you very far. You may just find yourself greatly disappointed when you fail to achieve your weight loss and health goals and consequently, ditch the whole thing.

So when you start fasting intermittently, always remember that it's all about synergy between its important components, i.e., fasting periods, feasting periods, timing, quality of food eaten, hydration, getting enough quality sleep, getting regular exercise and incorporating key practices into your lifestyle. When you look at the overall picture, you become less obsessed with each component and significantly increase your chances of sticking to your chosen protocol and achieve your weight loss and health goals.

A "Diet" Perspective

Lastly, the intermittent fasting practice isn't just a "diet" but a **lifestyle.** What this means is that it isn't something you just go all out on for a few weeks or months before ditching to go back to your previous eating habits. It's a way of life.

When you look at it from such a short-term perspective, you commit 2 other mistakes that can sabotage your efforts to achieve your desired body weight and good health. The first of these mistakes is that you may go to the extreme of being obsessed with intermittent fasting to the neglect of other important areas of your life like family, friends, and work, among others. Doing so can make you miss out on many of life's greatest joys and when you do, you may eventually blame intermittent fasting for it and ditch it altogether.

The second mistake that you may commit by looking at intermittent fasting as more of a diet rather than a healthy eating lifestyle is binge eating as soon as you're done with the diet. If you'll put everything on the line to go all out with intermittent fasting for a short period of time, you'll put yourself at high risk for recovering all the "lost eating opportunities" when you're done with it. And in most cases, people who binge eat right after dieting successfully tend to not only gain back the weight they lost but also add more pounds to their previously heavy weight.

When you look at intermittent fasting as a lifestyle, you will inadvertently consider all the other important aspects of a healthy lifestyle and increase your chances of not just fasting intermittently over the long haul but achieving your fitness and health goals.

Conclusion

As you've learned in this book, intermittent fasting is one of the best ways to get into great shape and good health. You also learned the different ways of fasting intermittently – a.k.a. protocols – and saw that regardless of your personal circumstances or schedule, you can incorporate it as part of your overall lifestyle. The only exception would be is if you have a pre-existing medical condition or special nutritional needs. But other than that, intermittent fasting can be a sustainable eating lifestyle that can contribute greatly to a fulfilling life.

But knowing is just half the battle of losing weight and achieving good health. The other half is action or application of knowledge. As such, I strongly encourage you to start applying what you learned in this book as soon as possible. And as I mentioned in some of the chapters, you neither have to apply everything all at once nor go cold turkey on food. Take baby steps and gradually build yourself up in terms of living the intermittent fasting lifestyle. By doing that, you significantly raise your chances of successfully incorporating it into your lifestyle and keep it there. And of course, you increase your chances of enjoying its key benefits – healthy weight loss and good health.

Here's to your success my friend! **Cheers!**

Please leave a review on Amazon if you found this book useful.!

CPSIA information can be obtained
at www.ICGtesting.com
Printed in the USA
BVHW040803250720
584657BV00015B/720